DATE: _____ W

Sleep (Hrs): _____

BREAKFAST	TIME:						
	TOTAL:						
	BLOOD SUGAR LOG:	Before/		After/		Insulin/	
SNACKS	TIME:						
	TOTAL:						
	BLOOD SUGAR LOG:	Before/		After/		Insulin/	
LUNCH	TIME:						
	TOTAL:						
	BLOOD SUGAR LOG:	Before/		After/		Insulin/	
SNACKS	TIME:						
	TOTAL:						
	BLOOD SUGAR LOG:	Before/		After/		Insulin/	

Water (Cups): _____

	Calories	Carbs (g)	Added Sugar (g)	Fiber (g)	Protein (g)	Fat (g)
DINNER TIME:						
TOTAL:						
BLOOD SUGAR LOG:	Before/		After/		Insulin/	
SNACKS TIME:						
TOTAL:						
BLOOD SUGAR LOG:	Before/		After/		Insulin/	

PHYSICAL ACTIVITY

Activity	Duration	Intensity	Cal/Burn

VITAMINS/SUPPLEMENTS

NOTES

DATE: _____ WEIGHT: _____

Sleep (Hrs): _____

	Calories	Carbs (g)	Added Sugar (g)	Fiber (g)	Protein (g)	Fat (g)
BREAKFAST TIME:						
TOTAL:						
BLOOD SUGAR LOG:	Before/		After/		Insulin/	
SNACKS TIME:						
TOTAL:						
BLOOD SUGAR LOG:	Before/		After/		Insulin/	
LUNCH TIME:						
TOTAL:						
BLOOD SUGAR LOG:	Before/		After/		Insulin/	
SNACKS TIME:						
TOTAL:						
BLOOD SUGAR LOG:	Before/		After/		Insulin/	

Water (Cups): _____

	Calories	Carbs (g)	Added Sugar (g)	Fiber (g)	Protein (g)	Fat (g)
DINNER TIME:						
TOTAL:						
BLOOD SUGAR LOG:	Before/		After/		Insulin/	
SNACKS TIME:						
TOTAL:						
BLOOD SUGAR LOG:	Before/		After/		Insulin/	

PHYSICAL ACTIVITY

Activity	Duration	Intensity	Cal/Burn

VITAMINS/SUPPLEMENTS

NOTES

DATE: _____ WEIGHT: _____

Sleep (Hrs): _____

	Calories	Carbs (g)	Added Sugar (g)	Fiber (g)	Protein (g)	Fat (g)
BREAKFAST TIME:						
TOTAL:						
BLOOD SUGAR LOG:	Before/		After/		Insulin/	
SNACKS TIME:						
TOTAL:						
BLOOD SUGAR LOG:	Before/		After/		Insulin/	
LUNCH TIME:						
TOTAL:						
BLOOD SUGAR LOG:	Before/		After/		Insulin/	
SNACKS TIME:						
TOTAL:						
BLOOD SUGAR LOG:	Before/		After/		Insulin/	

Water (Cups): _____

	Calories	Carbs (g)	Added Sugar (g)	Fiber (g)	Protein (g)	Fat (g)
DINNER **TIME:**						
TOTAL:						
BLOOD SUGAR LOG:	Before/		After/		Insulin/	
SNACKS **TIME:**						
TOTAL:						
BLOOD SUGAR LOG:	Before/		After/		Insulin/	

PHYSICAL ACTIVITY

Activity	Duration	Intensity	Cal/Burn

VITAMINS/SUPPLEMENTS

NOTES

DATE: _____ WEIGHT: _____

Sleep (Hrs): _____

	Calories	Carbs (g)	Added Sugar (g)	Fiber (g)	Protein (g)	Fat (g)
BREAKFAST TIME:						
TOTAL:						
BLOOD SUGAR LOG:	Before/		After/		Insulin/	
SNACKS TIME:						
TOTAL:						
BLOOD SUGAR LOG:	Before/		After/		Insulin/	
LUNCH TIME:						
TOTAL:						
BLOOD SUGAR LOG:	Before/		After/		Insulin/	
SNACKS TIME:						
TOTAL:						
BLOOD SUGAR LOG:	Before/		After/		Insulin/	

Water (Cups): _____

	Calories	Carbs (g)	Added Sugar (g)	Fiber (g)	Protein (g)	Fat (g)
DINNER **TIME:**						
TOTAL:						
BLOOD SUGAR LOG:	Before/		After/		Insulin/	
SNACKS **TIME:**						
TOTAL:						
BLOOD SUGAR LOG:	Before/		After/		Insulin/	

PHYSICAL ACTIVITY

Activity	Duration	Intensity	Cal/Burn

VITAMINS/SUPPLEMENTS

NOTES

DATE: _____ WEIGHT: _____

Sleep (Hrs): _____

	Calories	Carbs (g)	Added Sugar (g)	Fiber (g)	Protein (g)	Fat (g)
BREAKFAST TIME:						
TOTAL:						
BLOOD SUGAR LOG:	Before/		After/		Insulin/	
SNACKS TIME:						
TOTAL:						
BLOOD SUGAR LOG:	Before/		After/		Insulin/	
LUNCH TIME:						
TOTAL:						
BLOOD SUGAR LOG:	Before/		After/		Insulin/	
SNACKS TIME:						
TOTAL:						
BLOOD SUGAR LOG:	Before/		After/		Insulin/	

Water (Cups): _____

	Calories	Carbs (g)	Added Sugar (g)	Fiber (g)	Protein (g)	Fat (g)
DINNER TIME:						
TOTAL:						
BLOOD SUGAR LOG:	Before/		After/		Insulin/	
SNACKS TIME:						
TOTAL:						
BLOOD SUGAR LOG:	Before/		After/		Insulin/	

PHYSICAL ACTIVITY

Activity	Duration	Intensity	Cal/Burn

VITAMINS/SUPPLEMENTS

NOTES

DATE: _____ WEIGHT: _____

Sleep (Hrs): _____

	Calories	Carbs (g)	Added Sugar (g)	Fiber (g)	Protein (g)	Fat (g)
BREAKFAST TIME:						
TOTAL:						
BLOOD SUGAR LOG:	Before/		After/		Insulin/	
SNACKS TIME:						
TOTAL:						
BLOOD SUGAR LOG:	Before/		After/		Insulin/	
LUNCH TIME:						
TOTAL:						
BLOOD SUGAR LOG:	Before/		After/		Insulin/	
SNACKS TIME:						
TOTAL:						
BLOOD SUGAR LOG:	Before/		After/		Insulin/	

Water (Cups): _____

DINNER TIME:	Calories	Carbs (g)	Added Sugar (g)	Fiber (g)	Protein (g)	Fat (g)
TOTAL:						
BLOOD SUGAR LOG:	Before/		After/		Insulin/	

SNACKS TIME:						
TOTAL:						
BLOOD SUGAR LOG:	Before/		After/		Insulin/	

PHYSICAL ACTIVITY

Activity	Duration	Intensity	Cal/Burn

VITAMINS/SUPPLEMENTS

NOTES

DATE: _____ WEIGHT: _____

Sleep (Hrs): _____

	Calories	Carbs (g)	Added Sugar (g)	Fiber (g)	Protein (g)	Fat (g)
BREAKFAST TIME:						
TOTAL:						
BLOOD SUGAR LOG:	Before/		After/		Insulin/	
SNACKS TIME:						
TOTAL:						
BLOOD SUGAR LOG:	Before/		After/		Insulin/	
LUNCH TIME:						
TOTAL:						
BLOOD SUGAR LOG:	Before/		After/		Insulin/	
SNACKS TIME:						
TOTAL:						
BLOOD SUGAR LOG:	Before/		After/		Insulin/	

Water (Cups): _____

	Calories	Carbs (g)	Added Sugar (g)	Fiber (g)	Protein (g)	Fat (g)
DINNER TIME:						
TOTAL:						
BLOOD SUGAR LOG:	Before/		After/		Insulin/	
SNACKS TIME:						
TOTAL:						
BLOOD SUGAR LOG:	Before/		After/		Insulin/	

PHYSICAL ACTIVITY

Activity	Duration	Intensity	Cal/Burn

VITAMINS/SUPPLEMENTS

NOTES

DATE: _____ WEIGHT: _____

Sleep (Hrs): _____

	Calories	Carbs (g)	Added Sugar (g)	Fiber (g)	Protein (g)	Fat (g)
BREAKFAST TIME:						
TOTAL:						
BLOOD SUGAR LOG:	Before/		After/		Insulin/	
SNACKS TIME:						
TOTAL:						
BLOOD SUGAR LOG:	Before/		After/		Insulin/	
LUNCH TIME:						
TOTAL:						
BLOOD SUGAR LOG:	Before/		After/		Insulin/	
SNACKS TIME:						
TOTAL:						
BLOOD SUGAR LOG:	Before/		After/		Insulin/	

Water (Cups): _____

DINNER TIME:	Calories	Carbs (g)	Added Sugar (g)	Fiber (g)	Protein (g)	Fat (g)
TOTAL:						
BLOOD SUGAR LOG:	Before/		After/		Insulin/	

SNACKS TIME:						
TOTAL:						
BLOOD SUGAR LOG:	Before/		After/		Insulin/	

PHYSICAL ACTIVITY

Activity	Duration	Intensity	Cal/Burn

VITAMINS/SUPPLEMENTS

NOTES

DATE: _____ WEIGHT: _____

Sleep (Hrs): _____

	Calories	Carbs (g)	Added Sugar (g)	Fiber (g)	Protein (g)	Fat (g)
BREAKFAST TIME:						
TOTAL:						
BLOOD SUGAR LOG:	Before/		After/		Insulin/	
SNACKS TIME:						
TOTAL:						
BLOOD SUGAR LOG:	Before/		After/		Insulin/	
LUNCH TIME:						
TOTAL:						
BLOOD SUGAR LOG:	Before/		After/		Insulin/	
SNACKS TIME:						
TOTAL:						
BLOOD SUGAR LOG:	Before/		After/		Insulin/	

Water (Cups): _____

	Calories	Carbs (g)	Added Sugar (g)	Fiber (g)	Protein (g)	Fat (g)
DINNER TIME:						
TOTAL:						
BLOOD SUGAR LOG:	Before/		After/		Insulin/	
SNACKS TIME:						
TOTAL:						
BLOOD SUGAR LOG:	Before/		After/		Insulin/	

PHYSICAL ACTIVITY

Activity	Duration	Intensity	Cal/Burn

VITAMINS/SUPPLEMENTS

NOTES

DATE: _____ WEIGHT: _____

Sleep (Hrs): _____

	Calories	Carbs (g)	Added Sugar (g)	Fiber (g)	Protein (g)	Fat (g)
BREAKFAST TIME:						
TOTAL:						
BLOOD SUGAR LOG:	Before/		After/		Insulin/	
SNACKS TIME:						
TOTAL:						
BLOOD SUGAR LOG:	Before/		After/		Insulin/	
LUNCH TIME:						
TOTAL:						
BLOOD SUGAR LOG:	Before/		After/		Insulin/	
SNACKS TIME:						
TOTAL:						
BLOOD SUGAR LOG:	Before/		After/		Insulin/	

Water (Cups): _____

	Calories	Carbs (g)	Added Sugar (g)	Fiber (g)	Protein (g)	Fat (g)
DINNER TIME:						
TOTAL:						
BLOOD SUGAR LOG:	Before/		After/		Insulin/	
SNACKS TIME:						
TOTAL:						
BLOOD SUGAR LOG:	Before/		After/		Insulin/	

PHYSICAL ACTIVITY

Activity	Duration	Intensity	Cal/Burn

VITAMINS/SUPPLEMENTS

NOTES

DATE: _____ WEIGHT: _____

Sleep (Hrs): _____

	Calories	Carbs (g)	Added Sugar (g)	Fiber (g)	Protein (g)	Fat (g)
BREAKFAST TIME:						
TOTAL:						
BLOOD SUGAR LOG:	Before/		After/		Insulin/	
SNACKS TIME:						
TOTAL:						
BLOOD SUGAR LOG:	Before/		After/		Insulin/	
LUNCH TIME:						
TOTAL:						
BLOOD SUGAR LOG:	Before/		After/		Insulin/	
SNACKS TIME:						
TOTAL:						
BLOOD SUGAR LOG:	Before/		After/		Insulin/	

Water (Cups): _____

	Calories	Carbs (g)	Added Sugar (g)	Fiber (g)	Protein (g)	Fat (g)
DINNER TIME:						
TOTAL:						
BLOOD SUGAR LOG:	Before/		After/		Insulin/	
SNACKS TIME:						
TOTAL:						
BLOOD SUGAR LOG:	Before/		After/		Insulin/	

PHYSICAL ACTIVITY

Activity	Duration	Intensity	Cal/Burn

VITAMINS/SUPPLEMENTS

NOTES

DATE: _____ WEIGHT: _____

Sleep (Hrs): _____

	Calories	Carbs (g)	Added Sugar (g)	Fiber (g)	Protein (g)	Fat (g)
BREAKFAST **TIME:**						
TOTAL:						
BLOOD SUGAR LOG:	Before/		After/		Insulin/	
SNACKS **TIME:**						
TOTAL:						
BLOOD SUGAR LOG:	Before/		After/		Insulin/	
LUNCH **TIME:**						
TOTAL:						
BLOOD SUGAR LOG:	Before/		After/		Insulin/	
SNACKS **TIME:**						
TOTAL:						
BLOOD SUGAR LOG:	Before/		After/		Insulin/	

Water (Cups): _____

	Calories	Carbs (g)	Added Sugar (g)	Fiber (g)	Protein (g)	Fat (g)
DINNER TIME:						
TOTAL:						
BLOOD SUGAR LOG:	Before/		After/		Insulin/	
SNACKS TIME:						
TOTAL:						
BLOOD SUGAR LOG:	Before/		After/		Insulin/	

PHYSICAL ACTIVITY

Activity	Duration	Intensity	Cal/Burn

VITAMINS/SUPPLEMENTS

NOTES

DATE: _____ WEIGHT: _____

Sleep (Hrs): _____

	Calories	Carbs (g)	Added Sugar (g)	Fiber (g)	Protein (g)	Fat (g)
BREAKFAST TIME:						
TOTAL:						
BLOOD SUGAR LOG:	Before/		After/		Insulin/	
SNACKS TIME:						
TOTAL:						
BLOOD SUGAR LOG:	Before/		After/		Insulin/	
LUNCH TIME:						
TOTAL:						
BLOOD SUGAR LOG:	Before/		After/		Insulin/	
SNACKS TIME:						
TOTAL:						
BLOOD SUGAR LOG:	Before/		After/		Insulin/	

Water (Cups): _____

	Calories	Carbs (g)	Added Sugar (g)	Fiber (g)	Protein (g)	Fat (g)
DINNER **TIME:**						
TOTAL:						
BLOOD SUGAR LOG:	Before/		After/		Insulin/	
SNACKS **TIME:**						
TOTAL:						
BLOOD SUGAR LOG:	Before/		After/		Insulin/	

PHYSICAL ACTIVITY

Activity	Duration	Intensity	Cal/Burn

VITAMINS/SUPPLEMENTS

NOTES

DATE:_____ WEIGHT:_____

Sleep (Hrs): _____

	Calories	Carbs (g)	Added Sugar (g)	Fiber (g)	Protein (g)	Fat (g)
BREAKFAST TIME:						
TOTAL:						
BLOOD SUGAR LOG:	Before/		After/		Insulin/	
SNACKS TIME:						
TOTAL:						
BLOOD SUGAR LOG:	Before/		After/		Insulin/	
LUNCH TIME:						
TOTAL:						
BLOOD SUGAR LOG:	Before/		After/		Insulin/	
SNACKS TIME:						
TOTAL:						
BLOOD SUGAR LOG:	Before/		After/		Insulin/	

Water (Cups): _____

	Calories	Carbs (g)	Added Sugar (g)	Fiber (g)	Protein (g)	Fat (g)
DINNER **TIME:**						
TOTAL:						
BLOOD SUGAR LOG:	Before/		After/		Insulin/	
SNACKS **TIME:**						
TOTAL:						
BLOOD SUGAR LOG:	Before/		After/		Insulin/	

PHYSICAL ACTIVITY

Activity	Duration	Intensity	Cal/Burn

VITAMINS/SUPPLEMENTS

NOTES

DATE: _____ WEIGHT: _____

Sleep (Hrs): _____

	Calories	Carbs (g)	Added Sugar (g)	Fiber (g)	Protein (g)	Fat (g)
BREAKFAST TIME:						
TOTAL:						
BLOOD SUGAR LOG:	Before/		After/		Insulin/	
SNACKS TIME:						
TOTAL:						
BLOOD SUGAR LOG:	Before/		After/		Insulin/	
LUNCH TIME:						
TOTAL:						
BLOOD SUGAR LOG:	Before/		After/		Insulin/	
SNACKS TIME:						
TOTAL:						
BLOOD SUGAR LOG:	Before/		After/		Insulin/	

Water (Cups): _____

	Calories	Carbs (g)	Added Sugar (g)	Fiber (g)	Protein (g)	Fat (g)
DINNER TIME:						
TOTAL:						
BLOOD SUGAR LOG:	Before/		After/		Insulin/	
SNACKS TIME:						
TOTAL:						
BLOOD SUGAR LOG:	Before/		After/		Insulin/	

PHYSICAL ACTIVITY

Activity	Duration	Intensity	Cal/Burn

VITAMINS/SUPPLEMENTS

NOTES

DATE: _____ WEIGHT: _____

Sleep (Hrs): _____

	Calories	Carbs (g)	Added Sugar (g)	Fiber (g)	Protein (g)	Fat (g)
BREAKFAST TIME:						
TOTAL:						
BLOOD SUGAR LOG:	Before/		After/		Insulin/	
SNACKS TIME:						
TOTAL:						
BLOOD SUGAR LOG:	Before/		After/		Insulin/	
LUNCH TIME:						
TOTAL:						
BLOOD SUGAR LOG:	Before/		After/		Insulin/	
SNACKS TIME:						
TOTAL:						
BLOOD SUGAR LOG:	Before/		After/		Insulin/	

Water (Cups): _____

	Calories	Carbs (g)	Added Sugar (g)	Fiber (g)	Protein (g)	Fat (g)
DINNER **TIME:**						
TOTAL:						

BLOOD SUGAR LOG:	Before/	After/	Insulin/

	Calories	Carbs (g)	Added Sugar (g)	Fiber (g)	Protein (g)	Fat (g)
SNACKS **TIME:**						
TOTAL:						

BLOOD SUGAR LOG:	Before/	After/	Insulin/

PHYSICAL ACTIVITY

Activity	Duration	Intensity	Cal/Burn

VITAMINS/SUPPLEMENTS

NOTES

DATE: _____ WEIGHT: _____

Sleep (Hrs): _____

	Calories	Carbs (g)	Added Sugar (g)	Fiber (g)	Protein (g)	Fat (g)
BREAKFAST TIME:						
TOTAL:						
BLOOD SUGAR LOG:	Before/		After/		Insulin/	
SNACKS TIME:						
TOTAL:						
BLOOD SUGAR LOG:	Before/		After/		Insulin/	
LUNCH TIME:						
TOTAL:						
BLOOD SUGAR LOG:	Before/		After/		Insulin/	
SNACKS TIME:						
TOTAL:						
BLOOD SUGAR LOG:	Before/		After/		Insulin/	

Water (Cups): _____

DINNER	TIME:	Calories	Carbs (g)	Added Sugar (g)	Fiber (g)	Protein (g)	Fat (g)
	TOTAL:						
	BLOOD SUGAR LOG:	Before/		After/		Insulin/	

SNACKS	TIME:						
	TOTAL:						
	BLOOD SUGAR LOG:	Before/		After/		Insulin/	

PHYSICAL ACTIVITY

Activity	Duration	Intensity	Cal/Burn

VITAMINS/SUPPLEMENTS

NOTES

DATE:_____ WEIGHT: _____

Sleep (Hrs): _____

	Calories	Carbs (g)	Added Sugar (g)	Fiber (g)	Protein (g)	Fat (g)
BREAKFAST TIME:						
TOTAL:						
BLOOD SUGAR LOG:	Before/		After/		Insulin/	
SNACKS TIME:						
TOTAL:						
BLOOD SUGAR LOG:	Before/		After/		Insulin/	
LUNCH TIME:						
TOTAL:						
BLOOD SUGAR LOG:	Before/		After/		Insulin/	
SNACKS TIME:						
TOTAL:						
BLOOD SUGAR LOG:	Before/		After/		Insulin/	

Water (Cups): _____

	Calories	Carbs (g)	Added Sugar (g)	Fiber (g)	Protein (g)	Fat (g)
DINNER TIME:						
TOTAL:						
BLOOD SUGAR LOG:	Before/		After/		Insulin/	
SNACKS TIME:						
TOTAL:						
BLOOD SUGAR LOG:	Before/		After/		Insulin/	

PHYSICAL ACTIVITY

Activity	Duration	Intensity	Cal/Burn

VITAMINS/SUPPLEMENTS

NOTES

DATE: _____ WEIGHT: _____

Sleep (Hrs): _____

	Calories	Carbs (g)	Added Sugar (g)	Fiber (g)	Protein (g)	Fat (g)
BREAKFAST TIME:						
TOTAL:						
BLOOD SUGAR LOG:	Before/		After/		Insulin/	
SNACKS TIME:						
TOTAL:						
BLOOD SUGAR LOG:	Before/		After/		Insulin/	
LUNCH TIME:						
TOTAL:						
BLOOD SUGAR LOG:	Before/		After/		Insulin/	
SNACKS TIME:						
TOTAL:						
BLOOD SUGAR LOG:	Before/		After/		Insulin/	

Water (Cups): _____

	Calories	Carbs (g)	Added Sugar (g)	Fiber (g)	Protein (g)	Fat (g)
DINNER TIME:						
TOTAL:						
BLOOD SUGAR LOG:	Before/		After/		Insulin/	
SNACKS TIME:						
TOTAL:						
BLOOD SUGAR LOG:	Before/		After/		Insulin/	

PHYSICAL ACTIVITY

Activity	Duration	Intensity	Cal/Burn

VITAMINS/SUPPLEMENTS

NOTES

DATE: _____ WEIGHT: _____

Sleep (Hrs): _____

	Calories	Carbs (g)	Added Sugar (g)	Fiber (g)	Protein (g)	Fat (g)
BREAKFAST **TIME:**						
TOTAL:						
BLOOD SUGAR LOG:	Before/		After/		Insulin/	
SNACKS **TIME:**						
TOTAL:						
BLOOD SUGAR LOG:	Before/		After/		Insulin/	
LUNCH **TIME:**						
TOTAL:						
BLOOD SUGAR LOG:	Before/		After/		Insulin/	
SNACKS **TIME:**						
TOTAL:						
BLOOD SUGAR LOG:	Before/		After/		Insulin/	

Water (Cups): _____

	Calories	Carbs (g)	Added Sugar (g)	Fiber (g)	Protein (g)	Fat (g)
DINNER **TIME:**						
TOTAL:						
BLOOD SUGAR LOG:	Before/		After/		Insulin/	
SNACKS **TIME:**						
TOTAL:						
BLOOD SUGAR LOG:	Before/		After/		Insulin/	

PHYSICAL ACTIVITY

Activity	Duration	Intensity	Cal/Burn

VITAMINS/SUPPLEMENTS

NOTES

DATE: _____ WEIGHT: _____

Sleep (Hrs): _____

	Calories	Carbs (g)	Added Sugar (g)	Fiber (g)	Protein (g)	Fat (g)
BREAKFAST TIME:						
TOTAL:						
BLOOD SUGAR LOG:	Before/		After/		Insulin/	
SNACKS TIME:						
TOTAL:						
BLOOD SUGAR LOG:	Before/		After/		Insulin/	
LUNCH TIME:						
TOTAL:						
BLOOD SUGAR LOG:	Before/		After/		Insulin/	
SNACKS TIME:						
TOTAL:						
BLOOD SUGAR LOG:	Before/		After/		Insulin/	

Water (Cups): _____

	Calories	Carbs (g)	Added Sugar (g)	Fiber (g)	Protein (g)	Fat (g)
DINNER TIME:						
TOTAL:						
BLOOD SUGAR LOG:	Before/		After/		Insulin/	
SNACKS TIME:						
TOTAL:						
BLOOD SUGAR LOG:	Before/		After/		Insulin/	

PHYSICAL ACTIVITY

Activity	Duration	Intensity	Cal/Burn

VITAMINS/SUPPLEMENTS

NOTES

DATE: _____ WEIGHT: _____

Sleep (Hrs): _____

	Calories	Carbs (g)	Added Sugar (g)	Fiber (g)	Protein (g)	Fat (g)
BREAKFAST TIME:						
TOTAL:						
BLOOD SUGAR LOG:	Before/		After/		Insulin/	
SNACKS TIME:						
TOTAL:						
BLOOD SUGAR LOG:	Before/		After/		Insulin/	
LUNCH TIME:						
TOTAL:						
BLOOD SUGAR LOG:	Before/		After/		Insulin/	
SNACKS TIME:						
TOTAL:						
BLOOD SUGAR LOG:	Before/		After/		Insulin/	

Water (Cups): _____

	Calories	Carbs (g)	Added Sugar (g)	Fiber (g)	Protein (g)	Fat (g)
DINNER TIME:						
TOTAL:						
BLOOD SUGAR LOG:	Before/		After/		Insulin/	
SNACKS TIME:						
TOTAL:						
BLOOD SUGAR LOG:	Before/		After/		Insulin/	

PHYSICAL ACTIVITY

Activity	Duration	Intensity	Cal/Burn

VITAMINS/SUPPLEMENTS

NOTES

DATE: _____ WEIGHT: _____

Sleep (Hrs): _____

	Calories	Carbs (g)	Added Sugar (g)	Fiber (g)	Protein (g)	Fat (g)
BREAKFAST TIME:						
TOTAL:						
BLOOD SUGAR LOG:	Before/		After/		Insulin/	
SNACKS TIME:						
TOTAL:						
BLOOD SUGAR LOG:	Before/		After/		Insulin/	
LUNCH TIME:						
TOTAL:						
BLOOD SUGAR LOG:	Before/		After/		Insulin/	
SNACKS TIME:						
TOTAL:						
BLOOD SUGAR LOG:	Before/		After/		Insulin/	

Water (Cups): _____

DINNER	TIME:	Calories	Carbs (g)	Added Sugar (g)	Fiber (g)	Protein (g)	Fat (g)
	TOTAL:						
	BLOOD SUGAR LOG:	Before/		After/		Insulin/	
SNACKS	TIME:						
	TOTAL:						
	BLOOD SUGAR LOG:	Before/		After/		Insulin/	

PHYSICAL ACTIVITY

Activity	Duration	Intensity	Cal/Burn

VITAMINS/SUPPLEMENTS

NOTES

DATE: _____ WEIGHT: _____

Sleep (Hrs): _____

	Calories	Carbs (g)	Added Sugar (g)	Fiber (g)	Protein (g)	Fat (g)
BREAKFAST TIME:						
TOTAL:						
BLOOD SUGAR LOG:	Before/		After/		Insulin/	
SNACKS TIME:						
TOTAL:						
BLOOD SUGAR LOG:	Before/		After/		Insulin/	
LUNCH TIME:						
TOTAL:						
BLOOD SUGAR LOG:	Before/		After/		Insulin/	
SNACKS TIME:						
TOTAL:						
BLOOD SUGAR LOG:	Before/		After/		Insulin/	

Water (Cups): _____

	Calories	Carbs (g)	Added Sugar (g)	Fiber (g)	Protein (g)	Fat (g)
DINNER TIME:						
TOTAL:						
BLOOD SUGAR LOG:	Before/		After/		Insulin/	
SNACKS TIME:						
TOTAL:						
BLOOD SUGAR LOG:	Before/		After/		Insulin/	

PHYSICAL ACTIVITY

Activity	Duration	Intensity	Cal/Burn

VITAMINS/SUPPLEMENTS

NOTES

DATE: _____ WEIGHT: _____

Sleep (Hrs): _____

	Calories	Carbs (g)	Added Sugar (g)	Fiber (g)	Protein (g)	Fat (g)
BREAKFAST TIME:						
TOTAL:						
BLOOD SUGAR LOG:	Before/		After/		Insulin/	
SNACKS TIME:						
TOTAL:						
BLOOD SUGAR LOG:	Before/		After/		Insulin/	
LUNCH TIME:						
TOTAL:						
BLOOD SUGAR LOG:	Before/		After/		Insulin/	
SNACKS TIME:						
TOTAL:						
BLOOD SUGAR LOG:	Before/		After/		Insulin/	

Water (Cups): _____

	Calories	Carbs (g)	Added Sugar (g)	Fiber (g)	Protein (g)	Fat (g)
DINNER TIME:						
TOTAL:						
BLOOD SUGAR LOG:	Before/		After/		Insulin/	
SNACKS TIME:						
TOTAL:						
BLOOD SUGAR LOG:	Before/		After/		Insulin/	

PHYSICAL ACTIVITY

Activity	Duration	Intensity	Cal/Burn

VITAMINS/SUPPLEMENTS

NOTES

DATE: _____ WEIGHT: _____

Sleep (Hrs): _____

	Calories	Carbs (g)	Added Sugar (g)	Fiber (g)	Protein (g)	Fat (g)
BREAKFAST TIME:						
TOTAL:						
BLOOD SUGAR LOG:	Before/		After/		Insulin/	
SNACKS TIME:						
TOTAL:						
BLOOD SUGAR LOG:	Before/		After/		Insulin/	
LUNCH TIME:						
TOTAL:						
BLOOD SUGAR LOG:	Before/		After/		Insulin/	
SNACKS TIME:						
TOTAL:						
BLOOD SUGAR LOG:	Before/		After/		Insulin/	

Water (Cups): _____

	Calories	Carbs (g)	Added Sugar (g)	Fiber (g)	Protein (g)	Fat (g)
DINNER TIME:						
TOTAL:						
BLOOD SUGAR LOG:	Before/		After/		Insulin/	
SNACKS TIME:						
TOTAL:						
BLOOD SUGAR LOG:	Before/		After/		Insulin/	

PHYSICAL ACTIVITY

Activity	Duration	Intensity	Cal/Burn

VITAMINS/SUPPLEMENTS

NOTES

DATE: _____ WEIGHT: _____

Sleep (Hrs): _____

	Calories	Carbs (g)	Added Sugar (g)	Fiber (g)	Protein (g)	Fat (g)
BREAKFAST TIME:						
TOTAL:						
BLOOD SUGAR LOG:	Before/		After/		Insulin/	
SNACKS TIME:						
TOTAL:						
BLOOD SUGAR LOG:	Before/		After/		Insulin/	
LUNCH TIME:						
TOTAL:						
BLOOD SUGAR LOG:	Before/		After/		Insulin/	
SNACKS TIME:						
TOTAL:						
BLOOD SUGAR LOG:	Before/		After/		Insulin/	

Water (Cups): _____

DINNER TIME:	Calories	Carbs (g)	Added Sugar (g)	Fiber (g)	Protein (g)	Fat (g)
TOTAL:						
BLOOD SUGAR LOG:	Before/		After/		Insulin/	

SNACKS TIME:						
TOTAL:						
BLOOD SUGAR LOG:	Before/		After/		Insulin/	

PHYSICAL ACTIVITY

Activity	Duration	Intensity	Cal/Burn

VITAMINS/SUPPLEMENTS

NOTES

DATE: _____ WEIGHT: _____

Sleep (Hrs): _____

	Calories	Carbs (g)	Added Sugar (g)	Fiber (g)	Protein (g)	Fat (g)
BREAKFAST TIME:						
TOTAL:						
BLOOD SUGAR LOG:	Before/		After/		Insulin/	
SNACKS TIME:						
TOTAL:						
BLOOD SUGAR LOG:	Before/		After/		Insulin/	
LUNCH TIME:						
TOTAL:						
BLOOD SUGAR LOG:	Before/		After/		Insulin/	
SNACKS TIME:						
TOTAL:						
BLOOD SUGAR LOG:	Before/		After/		Insulin/	

Water (Cups): _____

	Calories	Carbs (g)	Added Sugar (g)	Fiber (g)	Protein (g)	Fat (g)
DINNER TIME:						
TOTAL:						
BLOOD SUGAR LOG:	Before/		After/		Insulin/	
SNACKS TIME:						
TOTAL:						
BLOOD SUGAR LOG:	Before/		After/		Insulin/	

PHYSICAL ACTIVITY

Activity	Duration	Intensity	Cal/Burn

VITAMINS/SUPPLEMENTS

NOTES

DATE: _____ WEIGHT: _____

Sleep (Hrs): _____

	Calories	Carbs (g)	Added Sugar (g)	Fiber (g)	Protein (g)	Fat (g)
BREAKFAST TIME:						
TOTAL:						
BLOOD SUGAR LOG:	Before/		After/		Insulin/	
SNACKS TIME:						
TOTAL:						
BLOOD SUGAR LOG:	Before/		After/		Insulin/	
LUNCH TIME:						
TOTAL:						
BLOOD SUGAR LOG:	Before/		After/		Insulin/	
SNACKS TIME:						
TOTAL:						
BLOOD SUGAR LOG:	Before/		After/		Insulin/	

Water (Cups): _____

	Calories	Carbs (g)	Added Sugar (g)	Fiber (g)	Protein (g)	Fat (g)
DINNER TIME:						
TOTAL:						
BLOOD SUGAR LOG:	Before/		After/		Insulin/	
SNACKS TIME:						
TOTAL:						
BLOOD SUGAR LOG:	Before/		After/		Insulin/	

PHYSICAL ACTIVITY

Activity	Duration	Intensity	Cal/Burn

VITAMINS/SUPPLEMENTS

NOTES

DATE: _____ WEIGHT: _____

Sleep (Hrs): _____

	Calories	Carbs (g)	Added Sugar (g)	Fiber (g)	Protein (g)	Fat (g)
BREAKFAST TIME:						
TOTAL:						
BLOOD SUGAR LOG:	Before/		After/		Insulin/	
SNACKS TIME:						
TOTAL:						
BLOOD SUGAR LOG:	Before/		After/		Insulin/	
LUNCH TIME:						
TOTAL:						
BLOOD SUGAR LOG:	Before/		After/		Insulin/	
SNACKS TIME:						
TOTAL:						
BLOOD SUGAR LOG:	Before/		After/		Insulin/	

Water (Cups): _____

	Calories	Carbs (g)	Added Sugar (g)	Fiber (g)	Protein (g)	Fat (g)
DINNER TIME:						
TOTAL:						
BLOOD SUGAR LOG:	Before/		After/		Insulin/	
SNACKS TIME:						
TOTAL:						
BLOOD SUGAR LOG:	Before/		After/		Insulin/	

PHYSICAL ACTIVITY

Activity	Duration	Intensity	Cal/Burn

VITAMINS/SUPPLEMENTS

NOTES

DATE: _____ WEIGHT: _____

Sleep (Hrs): _____

	Calories	Carbs (g)	Added Sugar (g)	Fiber (g)	Protein (g)	Fat (g)
BREAKFAST TIME:						
TOTAL:						
BLOOD SUGAR LOG:	Before/		After/		Insulin/	
SNACKS TIME:						
TOTAL:						
BLOOD SUGAR LOG:	Before/		After/		Insulin/	
LUNCH TIME:						
TOTAL:						
BLOOD SUGAR LOG:	Before/		After/		Insulin/	
SNACKS TIME:						
TOTAL:						
BLOOD SUGAR LOG:	Before/		After/		Insulin/	

Water (Cups): _____

	Calories	Carbs (g)	Added Sugar (g)	Fiber (g)	Protein (g)	Fat (g)
DINNER **TIME:**						
TOTAL:						
BLOOD SUGAR LOG:	Before/		After/		Insulin/	
SNACKS **TIME:**						
TOTAL:						
BLOOD SUGAR LOG:	Before/		After/		Insulin/	

PHYSICAL ACTIVITY

Activity	Duration	Intensity	Cal/Burn

VITAMINS/SUPPLEMENTS

NOTES

DATE: _____ WEIGHT: _____

Sleep (Hrs): _____

	Calories	Carbs (g)	Added Sugar (g)	Fiber (g)	Protein (g)	Fat (g)
BREAKFAST TIME:						
TOTAL:						
BLOOD SUGAR LOG:	Before/		After/		Insulin/	
SNACKS TIME:						
TOTAL:						
BLOOD SUGAR LOG:	Before/		After/		Insulin/	
LUNCH TIME:						
TOTAL:						
BLOOD SUGAR LOG:	Before/		After/		Insulin/	
SNACKS TIME:						
TOTAL:						
BLOOD SUGAR LOG:	Before/		After/		Insulin/	

Water (Cups): _____

	Calories	Carbs (g)	Added Sugar (g)	Fiber (g)	Protein (g)	Fat (g)
DINNER TIME:						
TOTAL:						
BLOOD SUGAR LOG:	Before/		After/		Insulin/	
SNACKS TIME:						
TOTAL:						
BLOOD SUGAR LOG:	Before/		After/		Insulin/	

PHYSICAL ACTIVITY

Activity	Duration	Intensity	Cal/Burn

VITAMINS/SUPPLEMENTS

NOTES

DATE: _____ WEIGHT: _____

Sleep (Hrs): _____

	Calories	Carbs (g)	Added Sugar (g)	Fiber (g)	Protein (g)	Fat (g)
BREAKFAST TIME:						
TOTAL:						
BLOOD SUGAR LOG: Before/		After/		Insulin/		
SNACKS TIME:						
TOTAL:						
BLOOD SUGAR LOG: Before/		After/		Insulin/		
LUNCH TIME:						
TOTAL:						
BLOOD SUGAR LOG: Before/		After/		Insulin/		
SNACKS TIME:						
TOTAL:						
BLOOD SUGAR LOG: Before/		After/		Insulin/		

Water (Cups): _____

DINNER TIME:	Calories	Carbs (g)	Added Sugar (g)	Fiber (g)	Protein (g)	Fat (g)
TOTAL:						
BLOOD SUGAR LOG:	Before/		After/		Insulin/	

SNACKS TIME:						
TOTAL:						
BLOOD SUGAR LOG:	Before/		After/		Insulin/	

PHYSICAL ACTIVITY

Activity	Duration	Intensity	Cal/Burn

VITAMINS/SUPPLEMENTS

NOTES

DATE: _____ WEIGHT: _____

Sleep (Hrs): _____

	Calories	Carbs (g)	Added Sugar (g)	Fiber (g)	Protein (g)	Fat (g)
BREAKFAST TIME:						
TOTAL:						
BLOOD SUGAR LOG:	Before/		After/		Insulin/	
SNACKS TIME:						
TOTAL:						
BLOOD SUGAR LOG:	Before/		After/		Insulin/	
LUNCH TIME:						
TOTAL:						
BLOOD SUGAR LOG:	Before/		After/		Insulin/	
SNACKS TIME:						
TOTAL:						
BLOOD SUGAR LOG:	Before/		After/		Insulin/	

Water (Cups): _____

DINNER TIME:	Calories	Carbs (g)	Added Sugar (g)	Fiber (g)	Protein (g)	Fat (g)
TOTAL:						
BLOOD SUGAR LOG:	Before/		After/		Insulin/	

SNACKS TIME:						
TOTAL:						
BLOOD SUGAR LOG:	Before/		After/		Insulin/	

PHYSICAL ACTIVITY

Activity	Duration	Intensity	Cal/Burn

VITAMINS/SUPPLEMENTS

NOTES

DATE: _____ WEIGHT: _____

Sleep (Hrs): _____

	Calories	Carbs (g)	Added Sugar (g)	Fiber (g)	Protein (g)	Fat (g)
BREAKFAST TIME:						
TOTAL:						
BLOOD SUGAR LOG:	Before/		After/		Insulin/	
SNACKS TIME:						
TOTAL:						
BLOOD SUGAR LOG:	Before/		After/		Insulin/	
LUNCH TIME:						
TOTAL:						
BLOOD SUGAR LOG:	Before/		After/		Insulin/	
SNACKS TIME:						
TOTAL:						
BLOOD SUGAR LOG:	Before/		After/		Insulin/	

Water (Cups): _____

DINNER TIME:	Calories	Carbs (g)	Added Sugar (g)	Fiber (g)	Protein (g)	Fat (g)
TOTAL:						
BLOOD SUGAR LOG:	Before/		After/		Insulin/	

SNACKS TIME:	Calories	Carbs (g)	Added Sugar (g)	Fiber (g)	Protein (g)	Fat (g)
TOTAL:						
BLOOD SUGAR LOG:	Before/		After/		Insulin/	

PHYSICAL ACTIVITY

Activity	Duration	Intensity	Cal/Burn

VITAMINS/SUPPLEMENTS

NOTES

DATE: _____ WEIGHT: _____

Sleep (Hrs): _____

	Calories	Carbs (g)	Added Sugar (g)	Fiber (g)	Protein (g)	Fat (g)
BREAKFAST TIME:						
TOTAL:						
BLOOD SUGAR LOG:	Before/		After/		Insulin/	
SNACKS TIME:						
TOTAL:						
BLOOD SUGAR LOG:	Before/		After/		Insulin/	
LUNCH TIME:						
TOTAL:						
BLOOD SUGAR LOG:	Before/		After/		Insulin/	
SNACKS TIME:						
TOTAL:						
BLOOD SUGAR LOG:	Before/		After/		Insulin/	

Water (Cups): _____

DINNER	TIME:	Calories	Carbs (g)	Added Sugar (g)	Fiber (g)	Protein (g)	Fat (g)
	TOTAL:						
	BLOOD SUGAR LOG:	Before/		After/		Insulin/	

SNACKS	TIME:						
	TOTAL:						
	BLOOD SUGAR LOG:	Before/		After/		Insulin/	

PHYSICAL ACTIVITY

Activity	Duration	Intensity	Cal/Burn

VITAMINS/SUPPLEMENTS

NOTES

DATE: _____ WEIGHT: _____

Sleep (Hrs): _____

	Calories	Carbs (g)	Added Sugar (g)	Fiber (g)	Protein (g)	Fat (g)
BREAKFAST TIME:						
TOTAL:						
BLOOD SUGAR LOG:	Before/		After/		Insulin/	
SNACKS TIME:						
TOTAL:						
BLOOD SUGAR LOG:	Before/		After/		Insulin/	
LUNCH TIME:						
TOTAL:						
BLOOD SUGAR LOG:	Before/		After/		Insulin/	
SNACKS TIME:						
TOTAL:						
BLOOD SUGAR LOG:	Before/		After/		Insulin/	

Water (Cups): _____

	Calories	Carbs (g)	Added Sugar (g)	Fiber (g)	Protein (g)	Fat (g)
DINNER TIME:						
TOTAL:						
BLOOD SUGAR LOG:	Before/		After/		Insulin/	
SNACKS TIME:						
TOTAL:						
BLOOD SUGAR LOG:	Before/		After/		Insulin/	

PHYSICAL ACTIVITY

Activity	Duration	Intensity	Cal/Burn

VITAMINS/SUPPLEMENTS

NOTES

DATE: _____ WEIGHT: _____

Sleep (Hrs): _____

	Calories	Carbs (g)	Added Sugar (g)	Fiber (g)	Protein (g)	Fat (g)
BREAKFAST TIME:						
TOTAL:						
BLOOD SUGAR LOG:	Before/		After/		Insulin/	
SNACKS TIME:						
TOTAL:						
BLOOD SUGAR LOG:	Before/		After/		Insulin/	
LUNCH TIME:						
TOTAL:						
BLOOD SUGAR LOG:	Before/		After/		Insulin/	
SNACKS TIME:						
TOTAL:						
BLOOD SUGAR LOG:	Before/		After/		Insulin/	

Water (Cups): _____

DINNER	TIME:	Calories	Carbs (g)	Added Sugar (g)	Fiber (g)	Protein (g)	Fat (g)
	TOTAL:						
	BLOOD SUGAR LOG:	Before/		After/		Insulin/	

SNACKS	TIME:						
	TOTAL:						
	BLOOD SUGAR LOG:	Before/		After/		Insulin/	

PHYSICAL ACTIVITY

Activity	Duration	Intensity	Cal/Burn

VITAMINS/SUPPLEMENTS

NOTES

DATE: _____ WEIGHT: _____

Sleep (Hrs): _____

	Calories	Carbs (g)	Added Sugar (g)	Fiber (g)	Protein (g)	Fat (g)
BREAKFAST TIME:						
TOTAL:						
BLOOD SUGAR LOG:	Before/		After/		Insulin/	
SNACKS TIME:						
TOTAL:						
BLOOD SUGAR LOG:	Before/		After/		Insulin/	
LUNCH TIME:						
TOTAL:						
BLOOD SUGAR LOG:	Before/		After/		Insulin/	
SNACKS TIME:						
TOTAL:						
BLOOD SUGAR LOG:	Before/		After/		Insulin/	

Water (Cups): _____

DINNER	TIME:	Calories	Carbs (g)	Added Sugar (g)	Fiber (g)	Protein (g)	Fat (g)
	TOTAL:						
	BLOOD SUGAR LOG:	Before/		After/		Insulin/	

SNACKS	TIME:						
	TOTAL:						
	BLOOD SUGAR LOG:	Before/		After/		Insulin/	

PHYSICAL ACTIVITY

Activity	Duration	Intensity	Cal/Burn

VITAMINS/SUPPLEMENTS

NOTES

DATE: _____ WEIGHT: _____

Sleep (Hrs): _____

	Calories	Carbs (g)	Added Sugar (g)	Fiber (g)	Protein (g)	Fat (g)
BREAKFAST TIME:						
TOTAL:						
BLOOD SUGAR LOG:	Before/		After/		Insulin/	
SNACKS TIME:						
TOTAL:						
BLOOD SUGAR LOG:	Before/		After/		Insulin/	
LUNCH TIME:						
TOTAL:						
BLOOD SUGAR LOG:	Before/		After/		Insulin/	
SNACKS TIME:						
TOTAL:						
BLOOD SUGAR LOG:	Before/		After/		Insulin/	

Water (Cups): _____

	Calories	Carbs (g)	Added Sugar (g)	Fiber (g)	Protein (g)	Fat (g)
DINNER TIME:						
TOTAL:						
BLOOD SUGAR LOG:	Before/		After/		Insulin/	
SNACKS TIME:						
TOTAL:						
BLOOD SUGAR LOG:	Before/		After/		Insulin/	

PHYSICAL ACTIVITY

Activity	Duration	Intensity	Cal/Burn

VITAMINS/SUPPLEMENTS

NOTES

DATE: _____ WEIGHT: _____

Sleep (Hrs): _____

	Calories	Carbs (g)	Added Sugar (g)	Fiber (g)	Protein (g)	Fat (g)
BREAKFAST TIME:						
TOTAL:						
BLOOD SUGAR LOG:	Before/		After/		Insulin/	
SNACKS TIME:						
TOTAL:						
BLOOD SUGAR LOG:	Before/		After/		Insulin/	
LUNCH TIME:						
TOTAL:						
BLOOD SUGAR LOG:	Before/		After/		Insulin/	
SNACKS TIME:						
TOTAL:						
BLOOD SUGAR LOG:	Before/		After/		Insulin/	

Water (Cups): _____

	Calories	Carbs (g)	Added Sugar (g)	Fiber (g)	Protein (g)	Fat (g)
DINNER **TIME:**						
TOTAL:						
BLOOD SUGAR LOG:	Before/		After/		Insulin/	
SNACKS **TIME:**						
TOTAL:						
BLOOD SUGAR LOG:	Before/		After/		Insulin/	

PHYSICAL ACTIVITY

Activity	Duration	Intensity	Cal/Burn

VITAMINS/SUPPLEMENTS

NOTES

DATE: _____ WEIGHT: _____

Sleep (Hrs): _____

	Calories	Carbs (g)	Added Sugar (g)	Fiber (g)	Protein (g)	Fat (g)
BREAKFAST TIME:						
TOTAL:						
BLOOD SUGAR LOG:	Before/		After/		Insulin/	
SNACKS TIME:						
TOTAL:						
BLOOD SUGAR LOG:	Before/		After/		Insulin/	
LUNCH TIME:						
TOTAL:						
BLOOD SUGAR LOG:	Before/		After/		Insulin/	
SNACKS TIME:						
TOTAL:						
BLOOD SUGAR LOG:	Before/		After/		Insulin/	

Water (Cups): _____

DINNER TIME:	Calories	Carbs (g)	Added Sugar (g)	Fiber (g)	Protein (g)	Fat (g)
TOTAL:						
BLOOD SUGAR LOG:	Before/		After/		Insulin/	

SNACKS TIME:						
TOTAL:						
BLOOD SUGAR LOG:	Before/		After/		Insulin/	

PHYSICAL ACTIVITY

Activity	Duration	Intensity	Cal/Burn

VITAMINS/SUPPLEMENTS

NOTES

DATE: _____ WEIGHT: _____

Sleep (Hrs): _____

	Calories	Carbs (g)	Added Sugar (g)	Fiber (g)	Protein (g)	Fat (g)
BREAKFAST TIME:						
TOTAL:						
BLOOD SUGAR LOG:	Before/		After/		Insulin/	
SNACKS TIME:						
TOTAL:						
BLOOD SUGAR LOG:	Before/		After/		Insulin/	
LUNCH TIME:						
TOTAL:						
BLOOD SUGAR LOG:	Before/		After/		Insulin/	
SNACKS TIME:						
TOTAL:						
BLOOD SUGAR LOG:	Before/		After/		Insulin/	

Water (Cups): _____

	Calories	Carbs (g)	Added Sugar (g)	Fiber (g)	Protein (g)	Fat (g)
DINNER TIME:						
TOTAL:						
BLOOD SUGAR LOG:	Before/		After/		Insulin/	
SNACKS TIME:						
TOTAL:						
BLOOD SUGAR LOG:	Before/		After/		Insulin/	

PHYSICAL ACTIVITY

Activity	Duration	Intensity	Cal/Burn

VITAMINS/SUPPLEMENTS

NOTES

DATE: _____ WEIGHT: _____

Sleep (Hrs): _____

	Calories	Carbs (g)	Added Sugar (g)	Fiber (g)	Protein (g)	Fat (g)
BREAKFAST TIME:						
TOTAL:						
BLOOD SUGAR LOG:	Before/		After/		Insulin/	
SNACKS TIME:						
TOTAL:						
BLOOD SUGAR LOG:	Before/		After/		Insulin/	
LUNCH TIME:						
TOTAL:						
BLOOD SUGAR LOG:	Before/		After/		Insulin/	
SNACKS TIME:						
TOTAL:						
BLOOD SUGAR LOG:	Before/		After/		Insulin/	

Water (Cups): _____

	Calories	Carbs (g)	Added Sugar (g)	Fiber (g)	Protein (g)	Fat (g)
DINNER TIME:						
TOTAL:						
BLOOD SUGAR LOG:	Before/		After/		Insulin/	
SNACKS TIME:						
TOTAL:						
BLOOD SUGAR LOG:	Before/		After/		Insulin/	

PHYSICAL ACTIVITY

Activity	Duration	Intensity	Cal/Burn

VITAMINS/SUPPLEMENTS

NOTES

DATE: _____ WEIGHT: _____

Sleep (Hrs): _____

	Calories	Carbs (g)	Added Sugar (g)	Fiber (g)	Protein (g)	Fat (g)
BREAKFAST TIME:						
TOTAL:						
BLOOD SUGAR LOG:	Before/		After/		Insulin/	
SNACKS TIME:						
TOTAL:						
BLOOD SUGAR LOG:	Before/		After/		Insulin/	
LUNCH TIME:						
TOTAL:						
BLOOD SUGAR LOG:	Before/		After/		Insulin/	
SNACKS TIME:						
TOTAL:						
BLOOD SUGAR LOG:	Before/		After/		Insulin/	

Water (Cups): _____

DINNER	TIME:	Calories	Carbs (g)	Added Sugar (g)	Fiber (g)	Protein (g)	Fat (g)
	TOTAL:						
	BLOOD SUGAR LOG:	Before/		After/		Insulin/	

SNACKS	TIME:						
	TOTAL:						
	BLOOD SUGAR LOG:	Before/		After/		Insulin/	

PHYSICAL ACTIVITY

Activity	Duration	Intensity	Cal/Burn

VITAMINS/SUPPLEMENTS

NOTES

DATE: _____ WEIGHT: _____

Sleep (Hrs): _____

	Calories	Carbs (g)	Added Sugar (g)	Fiber (g)	Protein (g)	Fat (g)
BREAKFAST TIME:						
TOTAL:						
BLOOD SUGAR LOG:	Before/		After/		Insulin/	
SNACKS TIME:						
TOTAL:						
BLOOD SUGAR LOG:	Before/		After/		Insulin/	
LUNCH TIME:						
TOTAL:						
BLOOD SUGAR LOG:	Before/		After/		Insulin/	
SNACKS TIME:						
TOTAL:						
BLOOD SUGAR LOG:	Before/		After/		Insulin/	

Water (Cups): _____

DINNER	TIME:	Calories	Carbs (g)	Added Sugar (g)	Fiber (g)	Protein (g)	Fat (g)
	TOTAL:						
	BLOOD SUGAR LOG:	Before/		After/		Insulin/	

SNACKS	TIME:						
	TOTAL:						
	BLOOD SUGAR LOG:	Before/		After/		Insulin/	

PHYSICAL ACTIVITY

Activity	Duration	Intensity	Cal/Burn

VITAMINS/SUPPLEMENTS

NOTES

DATE: _____ WEIGHT: _____

Sleep (Hrs): _____

	Calories	Carbs (g)	Added Sugar (g)	Fiber (g)	Protein (g)	Fat (g)
BREAKFAST TIME:						
TOTAL:						
BLOOD SUGAR LOG:	Before/		After/		Insulin/	
SNACKS TIME:						
TOTAL:						
BLOOD SUGAR LOG:	Before/		After/		Insulin/	
LUNCH TIME:						
TOTAL:						
BLOOD SUGAR LOG:	Before/		After/		Insulin/	
SNACKS TIME:						
TOTAL:						
BLOOD SUGAR LOG:	Before/		After/		Insulin/	

Water (Cups): _____

	Calories	Carbs (g)	Added Sugar (g)	Fiber (g)	Protein (g)	Fat (g)
DINNER TIME:						
TOTAL:						
BLOOD SUGAR LOG:	Before/		After/		Insulin/	
SNACKS TIME:						
TOTAL:						
BLOOD SUGAR LOG:	Before/		After/		Insulin/	

PHYSICAL ACTIVITY

Activity	Duration	Intensity	Cal/Burn

VITAMINS/SUPPLEMENTS

NOTES

DATE: _____ WEIGHT: _____

Sleep (Hrs): _____

	Calories	Carbs (g)	Added Sugar (g)	Fiber (g)	Protein (g)	Fat (g)
BREAKFAST TIME:						
TOTAL:						
BLOOD SUGAR LOG:	Before/		After/		Insulin/	
SNACKS TIME:						
TOTAL:						
BLOOD SUGAR LOG:	Before/		After/		Insulin/	
LUNCH TIME:						
TOTAL:						
BLOOD SUGAR LOG:	Before/		After/		Insulin/	
SNACKS TIME:						
TOTAL:						
BLOOD SUGAR LOG:	Before/		After/		Insulin/	

Water (Cups): _____

	Calories	Carbs (g)	Added Sugar (g)	Fiber (g)	Protein (g)	Fat (g)
DINNER **TIME:**						
TOTAL:						
BLOOD SUGAR LOG:	Before/		After/		Insulin/	
SNACKS **TIME:**						
TOTAL:						
BLOOD SUGAR LOG:	Before/		After/		Insulin/	

PHYSICAL ACTIVITY

Activity	Duration	Intensity	Cal/Burn

VITAMINS/SUPPLEMENTS

NOTES

DATE: _____ WEIGHT: _____

Sleep (Hrs): _____

	Calories	Carbs (g)	Added Sugar (g)	Fiber (g)	Protein (g)	Fat (g)
BREAKFAST TIME:						
TOTAL:						
BLOOD SUGAR LOG:	Before/		After/		Insulin/	
SNACKS TIME:						
TOTAL:						
BLOOD SUGAR LOG:	Before/		After/		Insulin/	
LUNCH TIME:						
TOTAL:						
BLOOD SUGAR LOG:	Before/		After/		Insulin/	
SNACKS TIME:						
TOTAL:						
BLOOD SUGAR LOG:	Before/		After/		Insulin/	

Water (Cups): _____

DINNER	TIME:	Calories	Carbs (g)	Added Sugar (g)	Fiber (g)	Protein (g)	Fat (g)
	TOTAL:						
	BLOOD SUGAR LOG:	Before/		After/		Insulin/	

SNACKS	TIME:						
	TOTAL:						
	BLOOD SUGAR LOG:	Before/		After/		Insulin/	

PHYSICAL ACTIVITY

Activity	Duration	Intensity	Cal/Burn

VITAMINS/SUPPLEMENTS

NOTES

DATE: _____ WEIGHT: _____

Sleep (Hrs): _____

	Calories	Carbs (g)	Added Sugar (g)	Fiber (g)	Protein (g)	Fat (g)
BREAKFAST TIME:						
TOTAL:						
BLOOD SUGAR LOG:	Before/		After/		Insulin/	
SNACKS TIME:						
TOTAL:						
BLOOD SUGAR LOG:	Before/		After/		Insulin/	
LUNCH TIME:						
TOTAL:						
BLOOD SUGAR LOG:	Before/		After/		Insulin/	
SNACKS TIME:						
TOTAL:						
BLOOD SUGAR LOG:	Before/		After/		Insulin/	

Water (Cups): _____

DINNER TIME:	Calories	Carbs (g)	Added Sugar (g)	Fiber (g)	Protein (g)	Fat (g)
TOTAL:						
BLOOD SUGAR LOG:	Before/		After/		Insulin/	

SNACKS TIME:						
TOTAL:						
BLOOD SUGAR LOG:	Before/		After/		Insulin/	

PHYSICAL ACTIVITY

Activity	Duration	Intensity	Cal/Burn

VITAMINS/SUPPLEMENTS

NOTES

DATE: _____ WEIGHT: _____

Sleep (Hrs): _____

	Calories	Carbs (g)	Added Sugar (g)	Fiber (g)	Protein (g)	Fat (g)
BREAKFAST TIME:						
TOTAL:						
BLOOD SUGAR LOG:	Before/		After/		Insulin/	
SNACKS TIME:						
TOTAL:						
BLOOD SUGAR LOG:	Before/		After/		Insulin/	
LUNCH TIME:						
TOTAL:						
BLOOD SUGAR LOG:	Before/		After/		Insulin/	
SNACKS TIME:						
TOTAL:						
BLOOD SUGAR LOG:	Before/		After/		Insulin/	

Water (Cups): _____

DINNER	TIME:	Calories	Carbs (g)	Added Sugar (g)	Fiber (g)	Protein (g)	Fat (g)
	TOTAL:						
	BLOOD SUGAR LOG:	Before/		After/		Insulin/	

SNACKS	TIME:						
	TOTAL:						
	BLOOD SUGAR LOG:	Before/		After/		Insulin/	

PHYSICAL ACTIVITY

Activity	Duration	Intensity	Cal/Burn

VITAMINS/SUPPLEMENTS

NOTES

DATE: _____ WEIGHT: _____

Sleep (Hrs): _____

	Calories	Carbs (g)	Added Sugar (g)	Fiber (g)	Protein (g)	Fat (g)
BREAKFAST TIME:						
TOTAL:						
BLOOD SUGAR LOG:	Before/		After/		Insulin/	
SNACKS TIME:						
TOTAL:						
BLOOD SUGAR LOG:	Before/		After/		Insulin/	
LUNCH TIME:						
TOTAL:						
BLOOD SUGAR LOG:	Before/		After/		Insulin/	
SNACKS TIME:						
TOTAL:						
BLOOD SUGAR LOG:	Before/		After/		Insulin/	

Water (Cups): _____

	Calories	Carbs (g)	Added Sugar (g)	Fiber (g)	Protein (g)	Fat (g)
DINNER TIME:						
TOTAL:						
BLOOD SUGAR LOG:	Before/		After/		Insulin/	
SNACKS TIME:						
TOTAL:						
BLOOD SUGAR LOG:	Before/		After/		Insulin/	

PHYSICAL ACTIVITY

Activity	Duration	Intensity	Cal/Burn

VITAMINS/SUPPLEMENTS

NOTES

DATE: _____ WEIGHT: _____

Sleep (Hrs): _____

	Calories	Carbs (g)	Added Sugar (g)	Fiber (g)	Protein (g)	Fat (g)
BREAKFAST TIME:						
TOTAL:						
BLOOD SUGAR LOG:	Before/		After/		Insulin/	
SNACKS TIME:						
TOTAL:						
BLOOD SUGAR LOG:	Before/		After/		Insulin/	
LUNCH TIME:						
TOTAL:						
BLOOD SUGAR LOG:	Before/		After/		Insulin/	
SNACKS TIME:						
TOTAL:						
BLOOD SUGAR LOG:	Before/		After/		Insulin/	

Water (Cups): _____

	Calories	Carbs (g)	Added Sugar (g)	Fiber (g)	Protein (g)	Fat (g)
DINNER TIME:						
TOTAL:						
BLOOD SUGAR LOG:	Before/		After/		Insulin/	
SNACKS TIME:						
TOTAL:						
BLOOD SUGAR LOG:	Before/		After/		Insulin/	

PHYSICAL ACTIVITY

Activity	Duration	Intensity	Cal/Burn

VITAMINS/SUPPLEMENTS

NOTES

DATE: _____ WEIGHT: _____

Sleep (Hrs): _____

	Calories	Carbs (g)	Added Sugar (g)	Fiber (g)	Protein (g)	Fat (g)
BREAKFAST TIME:						
TOTAL:						
BLOOD SUGAR LOG:	Before/		After/		Insulin/	
SNACKS TIME:						
TOTAL:						
BLOOD SUGAR LOG:	Before/		After/		Insulin/	
LUNCH TIME:						
TOTAL:						
BLOOD SUGAR LOG:	Before/		After/		Insulin/	
SNACKS TIME:						
TOTAL:						
BLOOD SUGAR LOG:	Before/		After/		Insulin/	

Water (Cups): _____

	Calories	Carbs (g)	Added Sugar (g)	Fiber (g)	Protein (g)	Fat (g)
DINNER TIME:						
TOTAL:						
BLOOD SUGAR LOG:	Before/		After/		Insulin/	
SNACKS TIME:						
TOTAL:						
BLOOD SUGAR LOG:	Before/		After/		Insulin/	

PHYSICAL ACTIVITY

Activity	Duration	Intensity	Cal/Burn

VITAMINS/SUPPLEMENTS

NOTES

©Dartan Creations Ltd.
www.blankbookbillionaire.com

Made in the USA
San Bernardino, CA
28 June 2018